S E X
SPIRIT
&
Y O U

Books by John-Roger

Awakening Into Light
Baraka
Blessings of Light
Buddha Consciousness
The Christ Within & The Disciples of Christ with the Cosmic Christ Calendar
The Consciousness of Soul
A Consciousness of Wealth
Divine Essence
Dream Voyages
Drugs
Dynamics of the Lower Self
Forgiveness: The Key to the Kingdom
God Is Your Partner
Inner Worlds of Meditation
The Journey of a Soul
Loving...Each Day
Manual on Using the Light
The Master Chohans of the Color Rays
Passage Into Spirit
The Path to Mastership
Possessions, Projections & Entities
The Power Within You
Psychic Protection
Q & A Journal from the Heart
Relationships – Love, Marriage and Spirit
Sex, Spirit & You
The Signs of the Times
The Sound Current
The Spiritual Family
The Spiritual Promise
Spiritual Warrior
The Tao of Spirit
Walking with the Lord
The Way Out Book
Wealth & Higher Consciousness

For further information, Please contact:
Mandeville Press
P.O. Box 513935
Los Angeles, CA 90051-1935
323/737-4055
soul@msia.org · www.mandevillepress.org

JOHN-ROGER

S E X
SPIRIT
&
Y O U

revised edition

MANDEVILLE PRESS
LOS ANGELES, CALIFORNIA

Published by Mandeville Press
P.O. Box 513935
Los Angeles, California 90051-1935
www.mandevillepress.org
email: jrbooks@msia.org

Visit us on the Web at www.mandevillepress.org

Printed in the United States of America
ISBN 1-893020-03-7

Library of Congress Catalog Number 99-66229

CONTENTS

1

INTRODUCTION

2

FACTORS OF SEXUALITY

3

SEXUAL EXPRESSIONS

4

THE LOVING RELATIONSHIP

1

INTRODUCTION

Levels of Consciousness

Life on planet Earth is a learning process, allowing you a wide variety of experiences on many levels, and more important, the opportunity to learn from your experiences.

There are five levels of consciousness which are called the lower, psychic, or "negative" worlds. These levels—the physical, astral or imaginative, causal or emotional, mental, and etheric or unconscious—are "negative" like the negative pole on a car battery; they are not negative in terms of being evil. For a car battery to work, you must have both the negative and positive polarities in a certain relationship to each other. The negative pole is valuable; it's necessary to complete the charge and to produce the power that makes the car function.

In a similar way, human beings must have a certain balance of positive and negative aspects in order to function here in the physical world. Without both positive and negative, humans wouldn't have bodies, nor would they function on this level. There are levels of consciousness within each person that relate to the negative realms of existence. The physical body relates to the physical realm; the imagination, to the astral realm; the emotions, to the causal realm; the thought processes, to the mental realm; and the unconscious, to the etheric realm. These five negative levels exist both inside and outside each person.

To balance the negative polarity, there is a positive level of consciousness, which is the Soul or Spirit of an individual. The Soul relates outwardly to the Soul realm, which is the first realm of pure, positive energy and Light. This realm and all realms above it form the positive pole of the battery. Without both the positive realms and the negative realms, the universe as we know it would be incomplete and unable to function.

Karma

When people are born on this planet, they come in with certain traits and abilities, and they have agreed to complete certain actions. Karma means action; it means a direction, a path that a person is going to fulfill. For example, some people may be born with great talent for music. They learn to play several instruments excellently, begin composing music at an early age, and achieve great success and personal fulfillment from their accomplishments. Part of their karma is to express themselves through music. Others may find their most fulfilling expression comes from marriage and raising children, which is likely part of their karmic fulfillment.

The earth has been called "the classroom of this universe." People are often brought together to learn from one another. Two people may come together with personalities that complement each other so that one completes the other; they share their energies and abilities. They may function better together than separately. Great learning and understanding can take place in this type of relationship. This type of relationship can be called karmic in the sense that each person is better able to fulfill his or her karma through that relationship.

Other people who are brought together to learn from one another may resist or misunderstand the process; they may see it as difficult or unpleasant. In this way, the word "karma" sometimes becomes associated with situations that seem bad. Karma is not bad; karma is action, learning, progression; often it is an opportunity for completion. It is your attitude toward karma that can make it seem either good or bad while you're going through it.

On a broader scale, each society has its own path of karmic fulfillment, which manifests as the rules of that society. The rules teach that certain aspects of human behavior are deemed right or wrong, good or bad. Acquired knowledge is handed down from one generation to another. Depending upon the society, education may be oral and informal or written and highly complex. A moral code, which can differ from society to society, is taught as "the truth" within each culture.

In any society, however, there are certain areas of human experience that cannot be taught. There is a great deal about love and the loving relationship between two people that can be demonstrated to a certain degree, but must be lived and experienced directly in order for it to be part of anyone's learning experience.

2

FACTORS OF SEXUALITY

Learn about Sexuality

Sex is an area that almost everybody on this planet will discover through direct experience. You can teach people that a hot coal will burn them by burning something else and letting them watch. From that vicarious experience, most people will learn never to burn themselves with a hot coal. You can teach people many things by example, but there are certain levels within us that demand expression and personal experience. The sexual expression is one of these levels.

It's a good feeling to realize that sex isn't dirty and that it's a natural process of the human body. It's an even greater feeling to realize that you were not born in sin and that there is nothing sinful about the sexual relationship.

I know a man who, while he was growing up and studying different religious doctrines, was told by many people that he was born in sin. He asked his parents to tell him how they felt at the time he was conceived. He said to his mother, "I want you to be honest with me. I want to know. Did you or didn't you want me? Prior to finding out that you were pregnant, what were you feeling? Were you hating my father? Was he hating you? Were you making up? What?"

His mother said, "Son, we probably had a perfect sex life. We really got along well together."

He said, "What does that mean?"

She said, "When he wanted sex, I wanted it. We didn't think we wanted any more children because it was during the depression; we already had two girls and a boy, and that was a nice family. But it was one of those cold nights when it was nice to cuddle up close." She told him a lot of little details. She said, "You know, we wrapped our feet around each other to get warm. His back was a little cold, so I cuddled up to it, and my back was a little cold, so he cuddled up to it. That felt good, so we kissed each other and told each other how much we loved each other. Then, when we were feeling really close, we had sex together."

The son asked, "Did you know that night that you had conceived me?" She said, "No, but it wouldn't have made any difference because it was so beautiful."

He asked, "What happened after you found out that you were pregnant?"

She said, "Well, I wasn't too sure how we were going to get along financially. Your father wondered about having four children. He wasn't making more than six or seven dollars a day, but he was so thankful that he had a job that he would have worked 20 hours a day so that his family could eat. And there you were, coming right along."

He asked, "Did you hate me? Was I born in sin?"

She said, "Oh, my goodness, no! You were loved from the first minute you were born."

He said, "Oh, you mean you loved me? You didn't just think I was a burden or a nuisance?"

She said, "No, son, but after you, I hoped I wouldn't have any more children because I didn't know how we could afford them. But we got one more. She was born years later."

After the son talked to his parents, he called his sister and said, "You were a mistake, honey. You weren't part of the family. I was the last of the family. You were a mistake."

She said, "I asked Mother and Dad, and I was the only one who wasn't a mistake. Mom told me she had seen one of her sisters who had a cute little baby and had said, 'Oh, I wish I could have one more child.' And she got her wish. She prayed to God and here I am. I am because God insisted, and that is not a mistake."

She was right; that was not a mistake. That was divine destiny. There truly are no mistakes on this planet as far as people are concerned. We are all here because we have a right to be here, regardless of what anybody says. We don't have to prove anything to anyone.

Sexuality and the Creative Imagination

Many of you do not know that the level of sexual expression and the level of creative expression reside extremely close together within the physical body. In your state of not knowing, you may become confused in your feelings. A level inside you seems to urge for sexual expression when it may, in reality, be an urge toward creative expression. It may seem to be saying, "Let's go have sexual intercourse," because that's the experience to which you have conditioned yourself. But it may really be saying, "Create; bring forth something new out of your own beingness." You may find that the sense of satisfaction that comes from sexual intercourse lasts for a relatively short time: a few days, or maybe a week. The fulfillment that comes from lifting into a higher level of creative expression lasts much longer.

Because the sexual and creative drives are close together, there are many misconceptions about them. A man once told me that the sex drive was the most important drive on this planet. I said, "No way; the imagination is."

He said, "Prove it."

I said, "Okay. How long does sexual intercourse last on the average?"

He said, "About 10 to 15 minutes."

I said, "And how long does a person think about this act before it happens?"

He said, "Maybe weeks or months."

I said, "Yes. Now... how long does the act last?"

He said, "Ah... I get it... the imagination is the most powerful force."

The imagination is the creative force. When you can harness it and start putting your mind where you want your mind to be and not where your sexual organs want it to be, then you are overcoming the flesh. This doesn't mean that you renounce sex and become celibate. It means that you put sex in proper perspective and use it as an expression and a fulfillment, rather than as the most important thing in this world.

Sexuality and Spirituality

Since sexual expression is a form of creativity, the creative urge toward the sexual relationship (the sex drive) and the creativity of Spirit reside close together in the same area in the body. It is like a band encircling the body from just above the navel to an area of the thighs about five to six inches below the buttocks. When people feel the surging of Spirit, they often translate this as being a sexual urge. So they release it sexually, but find that they do not always have fulfillment.

It is because the sexually creative drive and the spiritually creative drive are so close together that people can practice spiritual deceit and become the deceived. People may practice spiritual deceit on you only if you allow it.

Spiritual people can become well-known as "bedroom athletes," but this is not a compliment. It can be a misdirection and misappropriation of spiritual energy. The sexual relationship can be of a spiritual nature, and is a high form of sharing when done in loving and responsibility. Sexually seducing someone in the name of spirituality, however, is considered a spiritual crime. People who feel that they can lift the consciousness of another person through the sexual relationship had better be able to prove it to those who know the truth on the inner realms of Spirit, or they may find themselves coming back to clear those patterns of deceit and sexual abuse. If you enter into these actions of spiritual deceit, you will harvest what you sow. This is called "creating karma," or actions that must be balanced. You are held responsible for your actions. The price of being released from the cycle of reincarnation is eternal vigilance. I don't work with the type of yoga that is concerned with the lower centers of the body because the people practicing this type of yoga are reincarnating onto the planet. Through MSIA[1], I work with the Sound Current of God and of the Light, which is centered in the third or spiritual eye and higher.

---

[1] MSIA, The Movement of Spiritual Inner Awareness, is an organization teaching Soul Transcendence, which is becoming aware of oneself as a Soul and, more than that, as one with God.

If you draw a line from the middle of the forehead to the center back of the head, and another line from just above the right ear to just above the left ear, the point at which they intersect would be the approximate location of the third eye. It has three levels: the physical, the mental, and the spiritual. The lower part of the spiritual eye is involved with the physical level. People who have clairvoyant vision can see through this part of the third eye and can use this to their advantage. They may seduce you sexually in the name of spirituality; they can see your sexual weakness and know how to capitalize on it. Or they could use this ability in a positive way, helping someone find an occupation that benefits not only the person, but the whole community as well.

The middle range of the third eye is involved with the mental and the emotional levels. I include the emotional here because people do think emotionally at times. Those who can perceive the middle range may be able to use you to further their own ends, not by using you directly, but by using you indirectly to reach into other areas. On the positive side, they can see what might be going wrong and correct it.

I don't work with any of these aspects of the lower two-thirds of the spiritual eye. If you enter into these areas, you may enter into spiritual deceit and have to return to this physical world to clear that deceit; you could be opening yourself to things you may not want to handle.

If you do become involved on these lower levels and experience some confusion and difficulty as a result, don't go crying to your spiritual teacher. These are actions that you promoted, so you are responsible for balancing them. Ultimately, these actions are neither right nor wrong, and, ultimately, they will not block your spiritual growth. They might, however, delay your growth and will certainly block you from the knowledge of your spiritual progress in the invisible realms.

The misuse or abuse of sexual energies can lead you into areas of karma that can be difficult to resolve. I am not implying that you shouldn't get married and have a sexual relationship with your spouse or that the loving relationship between husband and wife can't be spiritual. The point is to be honest. If you're expressing lust, call it lust. If you simply feel sexy, call it that.

Be honest. If you say it's spiritual and it's not, you may be committing a spiritual crime. There is no way you can get away from it. You can fool the person you're with, and that person will probably not pick up anything detrimental except your negativity. They may eventually wish they'd never seen you, met you, or heard your name, however. That attitude can pull them back into relationship with you so the action can be balanced with neutrality, saying, "I love you very much, but we don't have to express it through sex."

The top part of the spiritual eye allows you to see the spiritual within the physical, to see God in humankind, to see the God image in each person you meet. The awakening of this part of the spiritual eye is part of the work done through MSIA.

When people who are spiritual feel the energy of Spirit coming in, they may misinterpret it as a sexual feeling. It can be difficult to differentiate between sexual and spiritual creativity. Often, people misinterpret this energy. MSIA teaches techniques for going within yourself to check the information that comes your way, to see whether or not that information is correct within your levels of beingness, and to recognize what is right for you in any given situation.

The spiritual thrust is up and out. The lift of energy is up through the body and out through the crown chakra, the energy center at the top of the head. The sexual energy releases through the reproductive area. These two energies often become so interwoven that the spiritual energy is released along with the sexual energy. That is negative creativity. It will hold you in the lower realms, in the physical world. When you feel the sexual drive building up, you can bring that energy up through the centers of the body. Feel the energy being released through the higher chakras instead of the lower ones. This is one way to use these creative energies to lift you into higher levels.

Sexual Fulfillment

Much of the fulfillment of sex results from balancing the positive and negative polarities of the man and woman. The man has greater positive polarity in his body; the woman has greater negative polarity in her body. This does not relate to good and bad; they are simply different frequencies. At the time of sexual intercourse, an electrochemical-magnetic charge takes place between the man and the woman. It is this charge that produces sensation. It's vital; it makes the battery go.

The man releases his relative negativity into the woman during sexual intercourse. The woman receives his negativity and then releases it during her menstrual period. During her menstrual period, she releases from her body that which is negative and will not bring forward new life. When a woman reaches menopause and can no longer release the energy a man shares during sexual intercourse through menstruation, then the relationship and her choice of a partner are even more important. With a wisely chosen partner, the act of sexual intercourse can be an expression of mutual upliftment toward God.

A woman should be able to release this negativity as easily as washing her face, but in our "civilized" society we have made natural processes more difficult than they should be. For example, some movies show women in childbirth screaming in agony. A young girl watching these movies may think, "I'm going to go through that?! Not on your life!" She creates a strong resistance to the whole process. Then, a few years later, she starts her period, which brings with it the potential of childbirth. She may get cramps all through the abdominal area and across the lower back every month. She may have a difficult time releasing the negativity.

When a woman has a history of blocking her creative flow and shutting off this area of expression by pushing the energy back down into the creative center, she may develop many problems related to her menstrual flow. She may release her negativity partially through the altered glandular functions of her body. She may also feel anxiety and apprehension at times. She may slam doors, explode for no apparent reason, and then walk away, finding that she feels a little better. It's more difficult to release the negativity when the normal channels are not available. It's interesting to note that when a woman is in the positive creative process of childbearing, she doesn't have her menstrual period.

The patterns of resistance and stubbornness that women sometimes enter into in regard to the creative process can also cause weight problems. As a woman expresses resistance, she pushes energy into the lower areas of creativity and reproduction. As the energy is pushed down, it attracts excess weight into that area, which is from just below the rib cage to the upper thighs. This weight can be hard to get off. Diet will help, and a change of attitude will help even more. If the attitude becomes one of acceptance, release, and flow, the weight will drop off and the cramps will also release.

A woman may gain weight just before her period and feel bloated and uncomfortable because the resistance pattern often increases irritation and negativity during this time. It's sometimes called false pregnancy; the menstrual cycle is altered so that the period doesn't come on time. She may fear she is pregnant. It's an age-old process. When her period comes, she feels so much better because that negativity has been released and the cycle is beginning again.

Many women's problems such as cramps, lower-back pains, weight gains, false pregnancies, and even hysterectomies can be lessened or eliminated altogether if a woman has a positive attitude of acceptance toward her body and its natural functions. Just knowing these things and working to change the expression to a more positive one can help tremendously. The first law of Spirit, acceptance, is also the first law of the physical body.

A man who does not release his negativity through the normal process of energy exchange with a woman may release his negativity in other ways. One way is through nervous energy, what we call "bumming around"—getting in the car and going here and there, just moving around a great deal. Masturbation is another release for him, in a sense. He may also release negativity by going through it and expressing it. He may release it through drug abuse or excessive drinking. Although all these things may help him to release negativity, they are not the most effective or desirable ways. Men who block their flow of creative energy will often develop prostate gland trouble and other problems related to the genital area.

Many problems that women and men have with their skin result from the fact that their creative energies are not flowing freely. Other symptoms also manifest when the creative energies are not allowed to flow. Note that this does not mean that you must have sex four times a week in order to have a healthy, well-functioning physical body. I am talking about the creative energies, which may be expressed in many ways. Primarily, your attitude is the key to whether your expression is positive and creative, or negative and contracting.

You can block the flow of energy from the creative part of the body through anger, guilt, desire for revenge, fear, misunderstandings, and so on. If, for whatever reason, the energy flow is shutting off, it will produce a block in the creative area, which will attract negative energy. Then you may find yourself putting on weight through the hip area, the buttocks, and the abdominal section. When you are expressing yourself in a positive flow of energy and direction, you will find the body automatically coming into greater balance.

As mentioned earlier, the creative and sexual energies reside close together in the creative center of the body. At times, you may experience the stirring of creativity by Spirit. Since this also moves the sensuality of the sexual organs, your mind may move to the fantasy or the reality of the sexual experience. Then you interpret the spiritual experience as the desire for sex, and you release it through a sexual relationship and don't feel fulfilled. You're left with the feeling that something is not quite right.

Some people know about this difference between the sex drive and the creative drive of Spirit; they know that these areas are closely related and that misinterpretation is possible. If you choose not to express sexually, then the creative energy can come up through the higher channels and be expressed in Spirit. However, there are various religious denominations advocating celibacy that have their own hospitals where their people go for psychiatric care; because of their misunderstandings about the nature of creativity and sexuality, there are malfunctions within their bodies. In trying to move into the spiritual through denying themselves on the creative level, they were creating more problems for themselves.

When the sexual drive is thwarted or produces guilt or unfulfillment, it reflexes back up into the stomach and intestinal areas and then up into the shoulder, neck, and facial areas. Muscle spasms can occur, the face may break out in acne, and parts of the neck may go out of place and cause pain. Feelings of guilt about sex can cause many things to happen.

Some couples have sexual intercourse, but the husband is not a lover; he's a machine, and he finishes his action before hers is complete. Then she has to finish her action by her own means, and she may feel guilty about it, all because he's not smart enough to love her as she needs to be loved.

It is important to be able to talk to your spouse about problems such as this and clear the action with one other. All of these actions are natural; there is nothing naughty or nasty about them. During sexual intercourse, two people are coming together in the closest relationship possible on the physical level. They owe it to themselves and to each other to come together with as much love and understanding as necessary to make the sexual experience a joyous and fulfilling one for both of them.

Sexual Cycles

The sexuality of both men and women operates in cycles. I think statistics indicate that a woman's cycle is about 28 days, although it can vary quite a bit from this. What many people don't know is that men have a cycle, too, which may vary from about 21 to 24 days. At various times during this cycle, a man will be more feminine than masculine in his action. Similarly, the woman will feel more masculine than feminine at certain times in her cycle. This is natural. At the time of his cycle when the man is less assertive, he may appear to be passive. He may feel like saying, "If you want to have sexual relations tonight, then you'd better get busy and get things started because, as far as I'm concerned, we can watch the late show or go to sleep and forget the whole thing." When the woman is in the passive part of her cycle she may say, "Not tonight, honey. I'm just not in the mood."

Being aware of these natural cycles is important for a couple. Much of the time, it seems as if the cycles don't match. More than likely, the man's period of assertiveness comes on just at the time of the woman's menstrual period, and she says, "Sorry, honey." Then about the time the woman is really ready to go, the man is at the end of his cycle. So he gets a six-pack of beer and watches television all night or says, "The guys and I are going out to shoot some pool. Don't wait up." This is the way it seems to go a great deal of the time.

These cycles within both the man and the woman can cause some interesting things to happen at the time a child is conceived. If a child is conceived while both the woman and the man are in their feminine period, the child will probably be a girl. If both the woman and the man are in the masculine or aggressive part of their cycles, the child will likely be a boy. If the woman is in her feminine cycle, and the man is in the masculine part of his cycle, there are a lot of possibilities.

They might produce a girl with characteristics society would label masculine. Or they might produce a boy who has feminine, sensitive characteristics. There are other possibilities, but the basic process is that there is an energy exchange between two people that produces a certain combination of electromagnetic force fields. The factors that go into shaping the destiny of a child are highly complex, and they are partly decided by the electro-chemical-magnetic frequencies of both parents at the time of conception.

The Three Selves

When a child is born on this planet, he or she comes in with three distinct levels of consciousness. The one that we're most aware of is the conscious self. That is the level that we function through during most of our daily lives because, for the most part, it is the conscious self that makes the decisions of our daily lives—the schools we attend, the jobs we choose, the quality of our work, the kind of car we drive, the people we choose for our friends, and so on. The conscious self is the "master of the ship."

There is another level that we call the high self. It can also be called the superconscious mind, the over self, or other names. This level is above the conscious self. It is aware of all that goes on, sees clearly the life path, and knows your destiny. The high self expresses feelings of great inspiration and love and has lofty

23

ideals of beauty, harmony, and joy. At different times throughout our lives, we can feel the influence of the high self.

The third level of consciousness exists below the level of the conscious self, and we call it the lower self or basic self. There is strong evidence of the lower self's presence and activity in people's life patterns. The lower self is sometimes more easily observed in the behavior of children, since the conscious self of a child is not as developed and directive as it will be later in life. The temper tantrums that a child expresses often come from the level of the lower self, which may say, "I hate you, Mommy. I hate you, Daddy. I wish you were dead." The child's conscious self probably does not feel this way, but the lower self sometimes does, and it will express those feelings.

We can see a similar sort of behavior pattern within adults. The lower self may no longer express through temper tantrums, but the pattern is similar. The lower self may feel slighted by something the boss said, or it may feel rejected because the spouse went to bed early. It starts feeling the pressure and pain of the environment, and it will do something to relieve that pressure. This can look like going out and getting drunk. The next day, the person wakes up with a hangover and wonders, "Why did I do that?" They look at what the boss said from a conscious point of view and realize that there was no slight intended; the boss was just being careless with words. They find out that their spouse was coming down with the flu and that no rejection was intended; they just didn't feel well.

The conscious self can understand the behavior of others, put it into proper perspective, and work with that knowledge. The lower self may feel the patterns of hurt and upset for a while, however. If something similar happens, it may move again into feelings of rejection, even though the conscious self recognizes that those feelings are not necessarily valid.

The lower self can have desires and preferences that are not in common with the conscious self, and this can cause some problems. If the conscious self likes to be slim, but the lower self loves the taste of chocolate and enjoys indulging in sweets, there can be difficulty. If the lower self relates to alcohol and likes the experience of drinking, while the conscious self is trying to function effectively in a job and family pattern, this can cause great difficulty.

The lower self can be very strong and willful; if the conscious self is not strong in its direction and purpose, the lower self can exert a great deal of control over the life pattern of the individual. In some unusual cases, it can take over and control the life pattern. Many people give in to their lower selves far too much of the time and allow them to make decisions that should be made by the conscious self.

The lower self, as well as the conscious self and the high self, expresses a masculine or feminine polarity.

If the polarity of the lower self is different from that of the physical body, this can cause some interesting patterns to occur. Remember that it is the exchange of energy between the man and woman that is important in the sexual relationship. If the woman has a male lower self and the man has a female lower self, they will be sexually compatible; the energy can flow freely and be exchanged. The chances are good that such a couple would not produce children, however, because the woman's male lower self would not feel receptive toward childbearing. Although the man's female basic might want children, he would be physically unable to fulfill that action himself.

If both the husband and the wife have male basic polarities or if both of them have female basic polarities, there will not be much energy flowing on the sexual level when they come together during sexual intercourse. There will be some, but there will be positive hitting against positive or negative hitting against negative, which can create disturbance unless that sexual expression is superseded by the love they have for each other on the higher levels. If the attraction is only sexual, they are likely to divorce quickly.

If the man's lower self is male and the woman's lower self is female and if there is also physical, emotional, mental, and spiritual love, there will be a positive exchange of energy. It will be very easy for conception to take place because both lower selves will probably be urging toward that fulfillment and completion.

Another thing to be considered is that there is a time within the woman's cycle when she is in readiness for pregnancy. Shortly before her menstrual period, she can become pregnant very easily. Immediately after her menstrual period, it's rather difficult for a woman to become pregnant, but case histories have shown that it's not impossible.

Birth Control

The characteristics of the woman's conscious self, and the polarity and characteristics of the woman's lower self determine the birth control method that is best for each woman. The method that is right for one woman may not be the method that is right for another. There are too many individual variables. What is important is the flow of energy between the man and the woman. If that flow is blocked for any reason, and the woman cannot give herself freely or receive his energy freely, she may experience great difficulty physically, emotionally, and very possibly mentally and spiritually. She may feel that she is just selling herself for rent, clothing, spending money, food, and so on. This is really what it amounts to if the love, sharing, and joy of being together and expressing together are missing.

A woman I know got mad at her husband and told me, "Well, he's seen the last of that."

I said, "What's 'that'?"

She said, "Don't play dumb with me. You know what's going on."

I said, "Well, you know, 'that' can represent a lot of things. Which 'that' are you referring to?"

She said, "The 'that' where I'm not going to give myself to him anymore."

I said, "Sexual intercourse."

She said yes.

I said, "Why don't you say it, or do those words disturb you? You know, there's nothing wrong in talking about these levels. Sex goes on; it's a pattern of nature, like dandruff and changing clothes and washing. If it weren't for sexual intercourse, none of us would be here. So, instead of putting it down, why don't you put it where it belongs? It's important, although it's not the only important thing happening on this level. It's nice to keep things in a realistic perspective."

I asked her, "Do you realize that the man, representing the positive polarity, and the woman, representing the negative polarity, must be charged in order to function effectively? Do you realize that this is important on many levels to the well-being of them both?"

She said, "I don't want any more children."

I said, "You have to decide that. I'm not involved in that action."

She said, "But you are right. I have to keep myself charged; it hurts me as much as it hurts him when I shut myself off."

I said, "Don't kid yourself."

She said, "You mean, he'd find another woman?"

I said, "Look, be realistic. Sex is often a mechanical process with a man. It releases tension from the body. It makes him feel good. He releases his negativity into the body of the woman, and then she releases it at the time of her menstrual period. It's just that simple, nine times out of ten."

I continued, "That other tenth, however, is vitally important because this is where the higher law supersedes the physical law. If a man and a woman share a spiritual love coming out of the positive realms, then it matters very little what they do on these other levels. The energy will be exchanged and the fulfillment will be there. When you are spiritually loving another human being, it matters very little what you do on any other level because the spiritual level is the most important. If that level is balanced, all other levels will come into balance."

Then I talked with her about her difficulty expressing sexually. Much of the problem seemed connected to her not wanting more children. Her fear of becoming pregnant was blocking her expression. A little while later, she told me she had decided to begin taking contraceptive pills.

When I saw her again, we talked, and I recognized that the pill was not effective for her. It was true that she was not pregnant and that a great deal of sexual activity was going on, but she was experiencing more anxiety, irritation, and difficulty than before. Her skin had broken out, she had gained weight, and other negative things were happening within her.

I said, "You need to change something."

She said, "What would you suggest?"

I asked, "Are you still taking birth control pills?"

She said yes.

I said, "That's fine, but those pills are contributing to your irritation."

She said, "What would you suggest?"

I said, "I suggest that some women take birth control pills for no longer than nine months at one time and then stay off of them for the next three months. Some women say, 'I've been feeling so well since I started taking birth control pills. My body feels better; I'm more balanced.' If that is your experience, my suggestion does not apply to you. You decide what's best for you."

This woman stopped taking the pill. I saw her two weeks later, and there was a calm and quiet with her. I said, "No more pills?"

She said, "The day we talked, I threw them all away. My husband is being careful." This is only fair. The months that the woman is not on the pill, the man can be careful. He can use prophylactics.

Another method of contraception is the intrauterine device, or I.U.D. The insertion of an I.U.D. into a woman can often be painful. A woman may feel upset over having such an object placed in her body. It can also be painful for her during sexual intercourse. Any of these things can cause tension to appear in her body, blocking her flow of energy and interfering in the exchange of energy during sexual intercourse. This tension comes out of the creative center of her body and can cause problems on various levels.

There are several things that determine whether or not an I.U.D. will be an effective contraceptive for a woman. If the woman's lower self has a male polarity, it will automatically start rejecting the I.U.D. The rejection may show up as a form of cervicitis or as a mucus or pus-like discharge, the cause of which may be difficult for the doctor to isolate. A male lower self will attempt to push out the I.U.D. It may throw the body into spasms that cause it to go through great pain and discomfort.

If the woman has a female lower self and the man has a male lower self, there will be little difficulty with an I.U.D. There will be a free flow of energy, which an I.U.D. will probably not disturb. This is one reason why some women think the I.U.D. is the only answer. Even if the presence of an I.U.D. is causing some discomfort, blocking to some degree the free flow of energy, it is possible that a woman will make it work for her because of the love she and the man express for each other on higher levels. There are so many variables to deal with. When the spiritual love is there, however, all other levels come into balance.

There are many other forms of birth control, and new ones are being continually developed for both men and women. The key is to find what works for both partners, and this can take some experimenting. Patience, honesty, and loving with the process can be a part of the joy of the relationship between two people.

3

SEXUAL
EXPRESSIONS

Morality

There are many different ways to express sexuality and many variations in sexual activity. None are necessarily good or bad. There is no morality in Spirit; in Spirit there are no right or wrong ways to express sexuality. Morality is an aspect of society. Humans decide their own morality.

This brings up the idea of sexual variants. I don't call anyone a pervert or deviate because that brings in the attitude of right and wrong. There are various ways to express sexuality, so there are many sexual variants. I'll give you the classical terms, and then I won't deal with classical terms anymore because they label and categorize things that are only expressions. For definition, some sexual variants are peeping Toms (voyeurs), sadists, masochists, nymphomaniacs, homosexuals, lesbians, heterosexuals (that's a variation, too, depending on who is observing), transvestites, hermaphrodites, pederasts, transsexuals, and those involved with fetishes. Spiritually, there is no morality in these areas. Through the lessons of negativity, however, we have put a morality onto these expressions. It's like being a child and being told that if you touch your reproductive area you'll go crazy. That's a lie or else everyone would be nuts.

When you get high enough above the negative (sexual, physical, emotional, mental) levels of the body, you can have spiritual liberation. In spiritual liberation, you can enjoy the lower levels with less chance of getting caught up in them. That does not give you any sort of license, however. You must always be judicious about your activities. Always. In the Soul level, there is no morality. Morality is a social custom; it's different in Southern California than it is in aboriginal tribes. What other people are socially accustomed to doing is not necessarily right behavior for you.

Promiscuity

Different sexual expressions produce different results, and some may be easier to handle than others. One result of a great deal of unselective sexual expression can be illness in the body, such as venereal disease. Another result can be the scattering of creative energy that could be channeled in a more positive direction. Yet another result might be confusion and a loss of identity because of receiving too many frequencies into the body.

The sexual relationship is a rapid way of mixing your frequencies with those of your partner. That is why it can be a rapid way to lose your own identity. You can become confused about who you are and lose your conscious direction. If you engage in a sexual relationship with someone who is also having sexual relations with others, you will receive not only that person's frequency but the frequencies and emotions of those with whom he or she has exchanged energies. You become the "garbage collector," and that can be hell. Then you may become so unsure of your identity and worth that you give up the dignity of your consciousness and allow the lower desire patterns of your nature to run your life.

Promiscuous sexual encounters can confuse you on many levels. Because sexual and spiritual creativity reside so close together, sexual activity can compromise the spirituality, leaving you even more open to pick up the frequency of the last person you encountered in sex. When people enter into great confusion— "I don't understand; I am confused; I don't know who I am"—it may be one of the indicators that they are being promiscuous.

Be careful about making a judgment, however, because it may be that they are growing rapidly in Spirit. Such total growth can also bring a form of confusion. When you are growing in a departmentalized way, you feel good about it because you can label what's happening and control it fairly well. When you are experiencing a total growth, a growth on all levels around and within you, you may experience a certain amount of confusion. When you go beyond your confusion and look back, you'll understand what has been going on.

If you're going to have a sexual relationship with someone, do yourself a favor and have it with the most enlightened person you can find. For example, if a man goes to the area where "sidewalk princesses" hold reign and enters into the entertainment, not knowing how many "princes" she has already entertained that evening, he may walk away with a great deal of discord and confusion in his beingness. If she has many frequencies around her, he may pick them up.

If a man is promiscuous for a period of time and then decides to settle down with one special woman, he may have a hard time because he has these other frequencies for comparison. Maybe his wife doesn't shower one night or forgets to use breath spray, or maybe the stockings have been hanging in the bathroom for two days. It doesn't take much; little things can turn him off, but he can learn to look past these areas to the Spirit within.

Remember that God dwells in essence within each person. If you go into the sexual action in lust, your partner may turn you away with confusion afterward. Loving someone does not necessarily mean that you look to him or her for fulfillment, but that you are both looking in the same direction. This is a key. If you both look in the same direction and then turn to look at each other for a moment, you can't really do anything wrong. Everything you do will be spiritually right. Then when you enter into sexual intercourse, you will experience your spiritual energies blending with the physical energies of the body.

If you look in the same direction and don't see the same things and then you look at each other, you will confuse yourselves spiritually. Then the sexual relationship may become one of deceit and lust, instead of spiritual love. The Bible tells us not to commit adultery. Part of that is not to adulterate the spiritual energies. Sexual promiscuity by either partner creates great difficulty.

It's best to be highly selective in the choice of your sexual partner and to be honest in your relationship. If it is just a lust relationship, be honest about that. You may still get the confusion of the various frequencies, but you won't experience guilt as well. If you enter into a sexual relationship in deceit and dishonesty, however, you will create a karmic indebtedness that may be difficult to handle. I hope you understand this; it's important.

I once counseled a woman who had built up great fantasies in the sexual area. When she saw men to whom she was attracted, she created fantasies that excited her emotionally and caused the erotic areas of her body to prepare for a sexual fulfillment that might not occur. This was really unrequited love, which can be frustrating. Over a period of time this frustration can be detrimental to the consciousness because the person walks around in confusion.

After working with this woman and helping her release the karma that produced all this, I received a phone call from her. She said, "I've lost my libido. I don't feel the things I used to feel. I don't feel alive."

I said, "Are you talking about your sex drive?"

She said yes.

I said, "Well, why don't you call it that? There's nothing wrong with the sex drive. It's very nice in its place."

This woman had tilted the balance so far in the direction of sexual relationships that she had indebted herself in the sexual, psychic, emotional, mental, and etheric areas. As this was being balanced, she was finding herself in a neutral state. This caused her concern, and she asked, "How long do I remain in this neutral state?"

I said, "Do you want to go back to those other feelings and experiences? Do you want to go back into those patterns?"

She said, "Oh, no."

I said, "This time is set aside for you so that you're not being pushed around by the creative energies that come from the lower part of your body, so that you can contemplate and lift yourself spiritually and bring your life into the order that it has been lacking all these years."

She said, "That's fine, but am I ever going to have a normal sex life again?"

I said, "I haven't the slightest idea what's normal for you. If 'normal' means having sex four times a day, I doubt that you're going to get that back."

She said, "It's difficult because I'm living with a man and not enjoying it."

I said, "Did you ever stop to think that your karma with that person might be over?"

She said, "Yes, I thought of that. But will I get back my sex drive?"

I said, "You have never lost your sex drive."

She was having difficulty understanding that the creativity she had been expressing as sexual intercourse was now being lifted into the spiritual and was moving away the things around her that had confused her. She said, "I do feel much better. I feel better physically, emotionally, and mentally, and I realize that I haven't been bothered for two months by those old fantasies and emotions. But yesterday, I started wondering why I wasn't having all those urges I used to have." With that, she had again set herself up in confusion, which was all a part of her growth and her learning.

When people feel their sexual urge backing off, they often think they're losing their abilities. So they rush out to see how many people will have sex with them, and then they can really enter into confusion.

People often ask me, "Who is it all right to have sex with?" My point of view is, "With anybody you want; you're doing it." Many people wonder if they're picking up karma from being involved this closely with another person. The answer is yes, there is an exchange of certain karmic things between two people who are sexually involved. People often tell me that they don't want to pick up karma, yet they still want to be involved in sexual activity with another human being, feeling that this is part of their expression in the world. My suggestion is to find someone with a very bright spiritual Light who is moving toward God so there won't be too much difficulty in the relationship.

The problem here is that so many people proclaim themselves holy: "Here I am, moving toward God. I really am spiritual." There is a lot of spiritual deceit going on, particularly on the word level. Give people time, however, and most of them will demonstrate by their actions where they are spiritually.

If the Traveler[2] is working with you in Spirit, what you do on these lower levels will not stop that spiritual work. You can suit yourself. Remember, however, that what you do may stop or delay your realization of the work that is going on in Spirit. The choices are yours. The Traveler doesn't care what you decide, because as long as you agree to work together

---

[2] The Traveler is a spiritual consciousness residing in every person. It is a guide into the higher levels of Spirit, the greater reality of God.

to release you into higher spiritual consciousness, then that's the work the Traveler does.

Prostitution

There is no need to label people or call them names. If you see a prostitute, you don't need to call her a dirty name. You don't know her karma or what's gone on in her life, so why label her? Maybe being a prostitute will help her complete her karma and free her from this level. If you judge her, you may find yourself experiencing that expression. It can be a rough life, but it is also just another level of expression.

Because prostitutes receive so many frequencies into their bodies, they have a tendency to lose track of who they are. One prostitute may receive five different frequencies into her body in one night. Then when she goes home and is with herself, she may come to the point where she says, "I am not worth a damn." That is a point of concern because she has denied the Spirit within her, which is expressing this way in order to bring her fulfillment of her karmic path. That denial is where the true concern lies.

A woman once came to me for a consultation. I talked with her about her life pattern and never once used the word prostitute. I knew she had been expressing this way, but there was no need to label her. After the consultation, she asked, "Why didn't you talk about prostitution?" I rewound a portion of the tape recording of the session and played it back to her. I said, "Now, all you have to do is substitute the word prostitution for these other words."

The woman said, "I thought you were talking about it, but I wasn't sure. I understand the karma of this action. When does the karma end?"

I said, "Right now, if you want."

She said, "You mean I don't have to do this anymore?"

I said, "No, no more."

When I saw the woman three weeks later, she told me she had a job as a secretary, and everything was fine. This was years ago, and I'm still working with her spiritually. If you met her, you would never know that she had at one time expressed prostitution.

Homosexuality

A man came for a consultation one day and said he was a confirmed homosexual. I said, "I'm not even sure I know what that is." He said that he found greater joy in men's bodies than in women's bodies. His fear was that he'd be fired from his job if his boss found out. I said, "Then why don't you tell him and see if he fires you? If he does, you can get another job where you'll be happier and won't be under so much pressure."

I explained to this man that his problem was not homosexuality, but his attitude toward it. He said, "But my psychiatrist says I'm sick."

I said, "Would you like to know how many homosexual psychiatrists, psychologists, and social workers there are in this area?"

I explained the karma of this action to him, which helped him to understand his experience. I told him that, in his situation, the karma was lifelong unless he could accept his position and not be concerned about what anybody thought about it. When he felt clear, he would have fulfilled his karma and it would be released.

This man had a whole pattern of lower-self responses: "The police will throw me in jail. What will the neighbors think? What will my mother think? I'm a man, but I feel feminine." I outlined these attitudes for him and said, "That is the part that's sick; nothing bad has happened, yet you've built up so much fear that you're running scared. You can't sit down and enjoy a cup of coffee for fear that someone will find out something that's within you."

The polarity balance of the lower self may partly determine a person's sexual preferences. If a man has a feminine lower self, particularly if that lower self is strong, he may feel a greater affinity for feminine things and be more comfortable expressing sexually with another man than with a woman. The same applies to a woman who has a lower self that is masculine. She may prefer to express sexually with another woman. A man with a masculine lower self or a woman with a feminine lower self may also express homosexuality; this will probably be a karmic situation with them.

45

Masturbation

When people are denied a natural sexual expression with a member of the opposite sex, they often misdirect their sexual energies to other forms of sexual expression, such as masturbation. In some monastic communities in Tibet or India, men live for years and never see a woman. There is a great deal of masturbation going on. This can be a negative expression because in masturbation, a person usually creates something in their mind that isn't real and then pretends it is, when nothing is actually taking place. Some men say, "I'm going to India or Tibet or China to become a holy man. I'm going to shave my head, wear saffron robes, renounce the world, and have no women around. Then I won't be tempted." Yet they will be tempted by the mind.

People who are astute and aware have seen that more than 70 percent of the people who deny themselves sexual expression with another person use their creativity, not in spiritual upliftment, but in self-gratification in the sexual area. Whom do they think they're kidding? What kind of game are they playing? They've released the energy for no purpose, to no avail. That energy will stay in their presence and cycle around on them the next night to be exercised again. With others, however, the image is, "I'm a holy man, holier than you." Yet that night they will again have difficulty fulfilling their levels of creativity and sexuality.

Sexual energy is extremely powerful. In masturbation, a tremendous energy is built up, and it cannot be released because there is no one there into whom it can be released. So it continues to build up and recycles.

Great thought forms can be created from the process of masturbation. These thought forms can be so large that they extend out from a person's physical body. This can be interpreted by others several ways: "He thinks he's the local stud" or "He thinks he's really a lady's man" or "There's a funny feeling I get from him, and I don't trust him" or "There's an animal quality with him."

This type of thought form can make it difficult for a man to have a fulfilling sexual relationship with one woman, so he may continue to add to the thought form the patterns of masturbation. He increasingly lets his lower levels of consciousness direct and run his life, making it more difficult for him to release his energies in a positive way. This creates a cycle that can be difficult to handle.

If a man masturbates often and then at some time decides to get married, he may find that the image he's created through his own sexual energies cannot be fulfilled by the woman. So he divorces her, picks up another woman, finds that she can't fulfill him either, divorces her, and so on. He may finally say, "I don't like women." Maybe all he can relate to is a magazine centerfold and his imagination. That's one way of expressing sexuality, but it is not the most positive way. A man's negativity cannot be effectively released through masturbation, so that negativity continually recycles, and that urge for release continues. It can be a very unfulfilling and unhappy situation.

Androgyny

Most of us are aware of bipolarity, of being either feminine or masculine. We can look at this objectively. In the past, one look was sufficient to identify anyone as male or female. Now, we see people whose bodies could be either male or female. Fashion trends have somewhat reflected this with the "unisex" look. Many clothing styles today can be worn by men or women.

Those who are androgynous often do not understand their nature and don't feel at ease in situations that seem normal to other people. People who are androgynous in nature need to have a balance within themselves. They do not necessarily need to come in contact with anyone else to achieve this balance; they can create it within themselves. If they are in balance within themselves, contact with strong positive or negative polarities can actually throw them out of balance.

When this happens, an androgynous person may react in several ways. One may be retreating through daydreaming, and another may be thinking, "What am I doing here?" or feeling a great discomfort with what's going on. Androgynous people often try to fit into a world designed for male and female polarities, into life the way it has been set up by society. They find that they don't fit and think, "My God, I don't fit in. How can I be here and not fit? I've got to fit, yet I'm a misfit." They may start grouping together and can represent an unusual cultural look. You might realize these people are different, yet be unable to identify what the difference is.

Many of these androgynous beings are bridging a gap between the present root race of the planet and a new root race that is coming in. The androgynous consciousness may be reflected more in attitudes and expression than in physical structure.

For the past 2,000 years or more, people have tried to become androgynous. An example would be a man and a woman who are married; the woman likes her "night out with the girls," and the man likes his "night out with the boys." This can be part of an age-old battle. The wife may say, "Why do you want to go out with your friends? Why don't you stay home with me?"

He says, "My God, honey, I wish I could tell you, but I just have to go out and have a beer, or shoot a game of pool, or maybe just stand around on the street corner and watch."

She says, "Watch what?"

He says, "I don't know. I haven't seen it yet."

Now she may get factious and say, "Yeah, watch the girls go by and then follow one."

Then he says, "That's not my intent." He doesn't know how to say, "My intent is part of this androgynous fulfillment" or "I must have male companionship." He probably has no understanding of this part of his nature. Nor is the woman aware that she must have female companionship because it's part of the androgynous fulfillment.

Androgynous people come together in both positive and negative balance and can flow in either direction. They express a polarity direction and can refuse to be bound by society's laws, which may be in direct opposition to what's going on inside them.

The androgynous consciousness is not yet the order of the day, but for many thousands of years the human consciousness has been moving in that direction. As we move further into the next age, we will be aware of more people expressing this way. Those people who do not yet have that consciousness, who are neither born into it nor learning to gravitate toward it, may find themselves at odds with the world. Such people may try to bring on a new "dark age" to try to hold things to a rigid point of view. Laws may become so strict that they are almost unbearable. If you think the old "spitting on the sidewalk" laws were strange, wait until you see the ones these people may try to create.

As more androgynous people come forward, they realize that they are not "this" and they are not "that."

They realize that they have a different reference point. They function in a center balance that is narrow compared to the opposite polarities of male and female. Within their scale they are very free, however. They will set up new forms of dress and new ways of expressing in the levels of morality. It will be the androgynous expression fulfilled. The new order of the day will be self-expression.

The androgynous consciousness is coming in to fulfill a new era. Many people who now have a bipolar consciousness may start moving toward androgyny, and this may cause confusion, uncertainty, and ambivalent feelings. The best thing anyone in this type of situation can do is just hang on and go through it. Rechemicalizations of the body may be taking place. Neuroenergies may be changing in the body. This can sometimes bring about violent outward manifestations or feelings of being unable to cope with these changes. This won't happen to everyone, but it certainly will happen to some.

People with androgynous consciousnesses may or may not feel an urge to express sexually. They probably will not need sexual expression, since they already possess a balance of positive and negative polarities. They may express sexually as a fulfillment on an emotional level, however. They may marry, have families, and be very comfortable in that experience; they may express in a heterosexual, homosexual, or bisexual way.

In the range of possible sexual expressions, androgynous people have as many possibilities as people of bipolarity. They also have the possibility of maintaining their own creative energy balance and using that energy to lift themselves into higher levels of consciousness. The person of male or female polarity can also do this, but it's easier for androgynous people to do, especially when they understand and learn to work with their own natures.

Cooperating With Your Sexual Expression

If you have a problem expressing sexually the way you want, you have a right to work through that, just the same as you have the right to work through jealousy, greed, or emotional problems if you experience those. If you have an illness, you have a right to work through that and achieve health. These things happen; they are steps in your progression. They are for your experience and learning. Then you move on to higher expressions.

Years ago, if you had a child with Downs syndrome, nobody knew it; if one of your children was mentally disturbed, you'd never tell. Remember Bo Radley in *To Kill a Mockingbird*? He was the "dumb" one, the "crazy" one who saved people's lives. He wasn't really crazy. He had some problems he was working through, one of which was how to relate to people in a way that they could understand.

That's all we're dealing with on these levels. If you are a man that we would call heterosexual, and another man comes up to you and says, "Let's go to bed," do you have to react and call him names? No. If you prefer not to express homosexually, just tell him that. If you go up to a woman and say, "Would you like to go to bed with me?" and she says, "No, I prefer not to," does she get a chance to call you all the dirty names you may have called that man? Sure, but are you that which she calls you? No. The morality of the physical level can block the spiritual flow. What you do and with whom you privately do it are your own business. It's the exchange of energy that is important.

4

THE LOVING
RELATIONSHIP

Resolving Misunderstandings

There are many areas of personal and loving relationships, as well as sexual expression, that can cause confusion, hurt, and unhappiness. Yet these same areas can be among the greatest sources of happiness, joy, and fulfillment.

You are told to love and cherish your home. How do you do that? How do you cherish your home when, perhaps, it has been shaken by an earthquake and the foundation has cracked? Were you thinking of your house? I am referring to your home, the place within you where your true self, the essence of your beingness, dwells.

You're thinking of the one you love because it's the place where the self of your loved one dwells. When you think of your loved one, however, do you think about the little areas of bad breath, dandruff, curlers in the hair, make-up left on overnight, and waking up with a grumpy disposition? These are some of the little things that can add up to incompatibility.

At one point you and your spouse were compatible, before you began to judge inaccurately. You knew better in the beginning. The reason you were attracted to the person you married or to the person you loved was not to change that person to something else. It was to love that person for him or herself. If you compromise that position, you've lost your marriage. Be strong. If you're an artist and your spouse married you because you do beautiful art work, and if your spouse wants you to stay home more often, then stay home and do beautiful art. Your spouse will love you.

Some people get married and start in with, "Don't do this and don't do that; you did this wrong." That is not why you get married. You don't marry to raise a husband or a wife. You marry because it is vital. You love your partner for what is vital within him or her. Then you try to change that vital thing into something nonvital. You're not going to love that thing that is nonvital; you're going to leave that person.

We're often too busy trying to either change people or please them. It's fine to get along with people, but, in doing that, don't sacrifice your divine heritage that you are here to fulfill. Marriage is a noble institution. If you're going to marry, marry somebody who can see and understand these things. Then, if you're late coming home, your spouse won't think you're out with somebody else. Marry somebody who can sit and talk with you in a way that you can understand.

Marry with the attitude that when something happens that is hard for your spouse to handle, you will hold firm with them. You don't say, "If you'd done it like I told you, this wouldn't have happened." Deal with what's going on, not with what you talked about last week. You might want to say, "You know what we talked about last week and the week before that and the week before that? This is another one, honey. These are connected. Maybe it's time for you to look because you may have a habit going against you."

Don't bring things up to people to point out their imperfection or your perfection; just bring up the possibility that some things can block people from receiving the greater health, wealth, and happiness that is coming to them. Then you can walk away and never say another word to them in that area, because it's their choice. If they weren't aware of the pattern, they may be thankful that you helped them become more aware. They may also say, "I know it now, but I just can't change it yet. Something inside is holding me." That's karma, and that's fine. You can help them get through it, not by judging the karma, but by cooperating with them and holding the Light for them. This is important when you are working with other people, especially with your spouse.

What should you do when you become hurt, upset, or out of balance? Some people say, "Let it all out and tell them what you think." Others say, "Keep it inside and suppress it; don't let them know. Overlook it. Forgive and forget." If you really can overlook, forgive, and forget, then I suggest this as your main course of action. If these things stay in your mind and emotions, however, then you have not really forgiven or forgotten. If you cannot wholly forgive and forget, you have to do something else.

You may try to ascertain people's motives for what they're doing, often attributing to them greater awareness than they have. They may be doing things without really knowing what they're doing. So, ask yourself a few questions: How important to you is the person who is doing this? Is this your loved one? If you really love that person, tell that person how you feel so that he or she can be aware of what you're experiencing.

If the love is reciprocated, you may decide that you want to work together through these levels of hurt and misunderstanding so that you can express the great love that you feel for each other. You may eventually decide that you want to enter into marriage or a permanent relationship, where you are committing your futures to each other. Then it's important to tell each other what's going on inside you, particularly if it is anything that will affect your future together.

This kind of communication can be done harmoniously. First of all, be considerate and loving.

You might cook that person's favorite food for them, rub their back, make sure they are comfortable, and help with the dishes. Then sit down and explain to your loved one that you have a point of view. Explain the way you've seen something, and admit that you're not sure if you've seen it accurately.

Ask for your spouse's help. An honest appeal for help is difficult to deny. When someone comes to me and asks for my help in clearing a situation, I usually look at the situation and endeavor to assist that person, even if I'm the one who has caused the irritation. When I have presented my point of view, they often find out that there was no need to be irritated.

When we understand the other person's point of view, we often find that they weren't aware that their actions were causing an irritation. When we find ourselves in this position of unknowingly irritating someone, we can simply change our actions. We all have the ability to change. If you want to change something, just do it. Wanting to change and being willing to change are the big keys.

Cooperation

If things aren't flowing well with you at home or in your relationships, the block is probably in you. Nervousness can often be telling you that you're out of line with what's happening. When people tell me they're nervous, I say, "Stop what you're doing."

They say, "Stop what I'm doing? That's a stupid answer."

I say, "All right, if you want to get more nervous, continue with what you're doing, and you'll find out what I'm talking about."

One married woman I counseled was having an affair, and it was making her very, very nervous. I suggested that she stop what she was doing. She stopped and later said, "It's marvelous. You're a magician. My nerves have cleared up."

Her husband came to me a short while later and said, "I'm very nervous. You cleared up my wife's nerves. I thought maybe you could do something for mine."

I said, "Why don't you stop what you're doing?" He had been having an affair, too, and decided to stop. In three weeks their nervousness was gone, they quit yelling at their children, the children started doing better in school, and they had a happy family. These people later found a spiritual direction, too.

Then one night they dropped by to see me. The husband said, "I want to clear something spiritually with my wife."

The wife said, "I have some things I want to clear, too."

I said, "Fine."

The husband looked me straight in the eye, and said, "Honey, I have something to tell you." He was talking to his wife, but he couldn't look at her. "I've had affairs while we've been married."

She looked like she'd like to give him a piece of her mind, but didn't. She just looked straight at me (I wasn't saying anything) and said, "Honey, I'm sure that every night you were with someone else, I must have been with someone, too."

He said, "You mean that you've been to bed with other men?"

She said, "Yes. Do you mean that you've been to bed with other women?"

He said yes.

She looked at me and said, "He must have picked lousy women."

I said, "How's that?"

She said, "He hasn't improved."

I just burst out laughing.

Then he said, "Well, those men you were with weren't winners, either." So they were even there.

Their marriage had been like this: They slept in twin beds. If she stubbed her toe on the way from her bed over to his bed before they made love, he'd say, "Oh, honey, did you stub your toe? Come here and let me love it." If she stubbed her toe on the way back to bed after they had made love, he'd say, "You clumsy fool." If it's really love, then it's love coming or going. That's where you have to keep this whole thing centered.

While we were talking, I saw them moving their hands out toward each other as they cleared a few more areas. She said, "Sometimes he has bad breath or body odor, and it turns me off when he wants to kiss me."

I said to the man, "Can you handle this?"

He said, "Sure, I can just brush my teeth or take a shower."

I said to him, "By the way, did you know about this before?"

He said, "No, this is the first time I've heard about it."

I said to her, "What else?"

She said, "He's too fast sexually for me."

I said, "Oh, that can be a problem," and I asked him, "Can you handle this?"

He said, "I don't know. How will I do it?"

I said, "Change your mental imagery. When you make love, you think ahead to conclusion; she doesn't. She goes step by step."

He asked how he could change this.

I said, "You're an architect. Why don't you design a house?"

He said, "Well, yeah, but I'd end up designing the bed first."

I said, "That may be all the time it takes to get her with you. It may take practice in order for you to find out who you're sharing with and who you're loving. It may take a little while. But for your sake, for her sake, and for God's sake, don't be afraid to communicate."

Then the husband said, "Okay, I know I've got bad breath and body odor, but does she have to come to bed with curlers in her hair and that stuff on her face?"

I said to her, "Can you handle that?"

She said, "Sure, I'll do all that at a different time. Or I can get up earlier in the morning to take care of my hair."

I said, "Okay, what else?"

He said, "She wears these funny pajamas to bed with a string that ties in the front. There I am under the covers, trying to untie the string, and she's put a double knot in it."

I know this sounds funny now, but it wasn't funny to them at the time. So I said, "What do you do in that situation?"

He said, "I just forget the whole thing and roll over and go to sleep."

I said to her, "What do you think about that?"

She said, "Well, if he'd just start untying the string first it would be okay, but he doesn't. He starts making love to me first, and then by the time he gets that untied, I'm ready to give up. I was trying to use that as a mechanism to slow him down so that by the time he got through with the knot, I'd be ready. But it didn't work too well."

He said, "Why didn't you tell me that? I was just being dumb and didn't know it."

I said to him, "Well, how can you handle this?"

He said, "I guess I can love her more tenderly, hold her, caress her, share the things of joy, the things of love, and make sure she's with me so the timing is right."

I said to her, "What will you do?"

She said, "I'll wear a shorty nightgown."

I said to him, "How about you?"

He said, "I won't wear anything at all."

She said, "Well, if you won't, I won't either."

It was beautiful to watch them come into a oneness. They had come in to talk about having had affairs; that had been cleared, and now they were down to the "tiddlywinks" of why people have affairs. It isn't the big things; it's these little things that keep building up because one partner won't get breath spray and say to the other, "Open your mouth, and I'll use some too."

You have a right to do this with the person you love, the one with whom you're going to share in close, personal relationship. You have a right to set it up well so that you'll both benefit from it—sexually, physically, emotionally, mentally, and spiritually. You'll eventually benefit from it financially, too, because your creativity will be flowing the way it should, into the world, creating and bringing in the things that you need.

When I saw those two reach out and take each other's hand, I said, "Please decide right now if there are any legal things you need to handle. Are you going to sue for adultery?"

They said no.

I said, "Okay, because it's a standoff. Anything else legal?"

She said, "Well, he already gives me the paycheck."

I said, "Are you going to continue giving her the paycheck?"

He said, "Yes, she handles the money better than I do. I'd be a fool if I didn't."

I said, "Okay, in other words, the legal things are behind you. If you can put all that behind you, why don't you just put all this other stuff behind you, too?"

He said, "And the kids. Where do you think we could put them for a weekend?"

I said, "What?"

He said, "Where can we put the kids? When we leave here, we're going on a honeymoon. When we were first married, we were so together; and if we could do it then, we can do it now. But what do we do with three kids?"

I said, "Put them in the room down the hall."

They had their honeymoon and the kids went along.

When you are attempting to evolve a successful relationship with another person, that person may think you're trying to change him or her—and there's no need to lie and say you're not, because you certainly may be. You can say, "This may look like I'm trying to change you. I am trying to change something because I'm really uncomfortable with the situation. If we can change my point of view, that may be all that's necessary. If we can't, then before this gets to be a knock-down, drag-out fight, maybe we should get a third party to see if they can assist us."

People sometimes come up with the conclusion that they are just not going to see eye-to-eye with one another, which means their future together is over and they go their separate ways. I'm not recommending that people break up; I'm saying that it may happen unless each person can compromise and is willing to say, "Let's work together to change this."

Emotional Responsibility

Many people live in their emotions and express themselves through this level. Some people say "I think" when they really mean "I feel." We're on a "feeling" planet; it is through feelings that we reach out to people much of the time.

There comes a time for most people when they will make decisions that will be adverse to someone else's emotions. For example, a young man grows up in a family, goes to high school, and meets a young woman whom he wants to date. Her social status (or some other criterion) is different from that of his family or from the way his family sees itself. If he takes her out, not too much is said, but if they decide to go steady, they will bring a little discord into the family. That decision will be adverse to the rest of the family.

People know when their actions are creating this type of disturbance. If they can handle it, that's fine. It might be wise, however, to listen to the family's point of view, compare it with other points of view, and then make a decision based upon an intelligent evaluation rather than on emotional factors.

I used to do a great deal of premarital counseling. I did an analysis of each person and then let them see for themselves what the situation was. We would sometimes find that the attitudes of the two were so far apart that the marriage might come to an end within a short time. I'd suggest that before marriage, before they invested themselves emotionally or financially in each other and before they had a family on the way, they take a good look. It's easier to make the decision beforehand than to wait a few years when there might be children and extended family who would be affected. As a counselor I remained neutral. I kept my feelings out of it, and I didn't care if they got together or not. These couples would often say to me, "You really don't care one way or the other. Our parents care and are trying to influence us, and our friends care and are also trying to influence us. But you aren't trying to influence us one way or the other on anything."

My caring was that they make the best possible decision for themselves, the decision that would bring them the greatest happiness.

Many times the two would decide to go their own ways, eventually marrying different people after looking for someone who could work well with their personalities and values. I still hear from some of these people, who tell me that the reason they keep in touch with me is because I'm neutral. In that neutrality, people can see more clearly what they're doing and can make decisions that are supportive of themselves and others. This approach usually creates less adversity and more happiness for everyone involved.

Let's go back to the earlier example of the young man who is dating the young woman. If he continues to date her and they decide to marry, there may be tremendous discord between him and his parents. People can always see precisely, without any reservations, what another person should do with his or her life, even if they are having difficulty with their own. Parents often speak from such a position of authority, saying, "I'm older than you. I know better."

In this situation, a wise son or daughter says, "When I look at your life, I find I had better not listen to what you say because you're continually making errors in your decisions. I love you very much, but that's the way it is. You've raised me to think for myself. I can make decisions. I can see where things are out of balance and can then change my mind and make a more accurate decision. I can learn from my errors and mistakes."

Many parents won't recognize these abilities in their children. They say, "I'm your parent; you'll do as I say." Parents do not have this right. When they assert this type of authority, they cause a "generation gap" in the family, having forgotten that wisdom is not confined to any age bracket. Wisdom is where you find it, and truth is where you find it.

Each person must choose for himself or herself. There is no need to try to influence someone one way or another, but you can be honest and present different options and points of view. You can describe the possible results of various actions. You can lay out four or five choices. Then, whatever the person chooses will be all right with you because your emotions and ego won't be involved.

If you present only one choice, you'll usually find that your emotions and ego become involved, and you may try to control the person's decision. Then if the person decides against your recommendation, you could feel hurt, upset, and confused. When people feel this type of control from you, they will fight back. They'll say, "I love you, but let me breathe my own air." They may feel suffocated in many ways.

When you can look at a person and say, "I love you; do as you please," that person can say, "That's right! I'm free. I don't have to prove it to anybody. I love you, too, and you can do what you want to do." In that freedom, you may decide to go on together.

We can look at a man and a woman as being like an oak tree and a pine tree; neither one can grow in the other's shadow. Each must be far enough away from the other to send down strong roots. Those roots may mingle at the bottom, and when the trees grow tall, their branches may touch and become interwoven, but each one is bringing a distinct, powerful action that brings them together in harmony.

That action is one of saying, "Don't change for me, for you can never please me. If you change, change because you want to please yourself. Allow me the freedom to change as I want, so that I can please myself." When you make that decision to please yourself, you're happy. Then that happiness will bubble over to the people around you, and you'll say, "I feel so good. Let me scratch your back. Let me fix that for you. Let me do something for you." When you're feeling miserable, you say, "Go fix it yourself. Leave me alone. I've got a headache. My back hurts. I'm tired."

Taking care of yourself is a form of selfishness, positive selfishness. If you take care of yourself first, you can then take so much better care of those you love. If you sacrifice yourself, however, how can you help anyone else?

For example, I know a beautiful woman who dearly loves her family. She has seven children, and when they were all very young, they all got chicken pox, and then they all got the mumps. It was one of those years when the kids were picking up everything. The mother so loved the family that she stayed up night after night. The kids were itching, scratching, and crying, and she was up trying to make them comfortable.

During the daytime her husband had a certain demand on her time. When it was suggested to her that she get some rest, she said, "I can't rest. What if my children need me?" She was told, "It could be difficult on them if you aren't more careful." She could not accept that idea, and a short time later she went into the hospital with physical, mental, and emotional exhaustion. She didn't have a breakdown; she was just exhausted.

They had to bring in two nurses to finish taking care of the children. There were bills for the children's nurses, for the hospital, and for a nurse to take care of the mother during her recovery period. Because she didn't take care of herself, she couldn't take care of her family, and they didn't appreciate it when she wasn't there.

The kids told her in their own way, "Why didn't you take care of yourself? We worried about you when you were in the hospital and we were trying to get well. We wondered if you were sick, if you might die, if you'd come home and be all right again." The kids lay in bed and cried because she wasn't there when they needed her. She said, "How could I have been so stupid not to see?" We sometimes forget that if we don't take care of ourselves so that we can be self sustaining, we can't be of much assistance to anyone else.

If we're upset and confused, we're going to force our upset and confusion on somebody else. If two people are married and one has an emotional hang-up, that person may cause the other one emotional confusion, and then the marriage will be crippled. The existence will be crippled. If someone around you is emotionally upset, tell that person not to put that on you. You can help that person work through it, but don't take that confusion and upset on yourself. You don't have to allow that. Be selfish in a positive way.

You can enter into a consciousness of sacrifice, sacrifice, sacrifice. If that works for you, go ahead and do it. If you find, however, that your sacrifice makes you irritable and upset, then perhaps it's not working for you. If you start resenting those for whom you're sacrificing, then you can't really love them. You will be upset with every choice they make, and they'll be upset with every choice you make. At some point, you're going to have to back off and say, "Look, you're an intelligent person; you know how to make choices. You know what my feelings are. I've told you. Now you can make your own decision."

You may sometimes experience such a tremendous loneliness that no matter where you turn, there is only loneliness. So you say to your loved one, "You're not making me happy. I'm very unhappy." Your loved one may say, "That's your problem. You handle it." Then you're really upset. The fact is, however, that it is your problem to handle. Your loved one may not have said it as a put-down, but as a statement of fact and as a sincere suggestion: handle it. You can handle it because you know what can make you happy.

Generally, what makes a person happy? Consciously thinking about happy things. That's one way to define happiness. When you think of happy things, you direct your mind into positive areas. What is the happiest thing you can think of? Having understanding with someone and having them understand you? No, that's not enough. You must let your loved ones be responsible for themselves. You must trust that they can learn, that they can understand, that they can grow. And that's not enough either. You have to enthusiastically say, "Yes, go ahead, do it your way. It's fine" And you have to mean it. Instead, people too often say, "You can do it, I guess, if you really want to. But don't expect me to be here when you get back." That leaves the other person thinking, "You don't really trust me. You won't let me be responsible. You don't understand me. You don't love me."

It can get to the point where your spouse tells you this, and you hit at them in response. Then they know you don't love them, and that may not be true at all. It's just the way feelings and thoughts work sometimes.

When you feel this type of emotional hurt, you usually find it difficult to look deeply into the other person and see the beauty there. You must go past the physical imperfections, their scratching their nose in public, wearing mismatched socks, or using poor grammar. These are little things that are imperfect and that may never be perfect. These little things can mount up to great big things that you can never resolve because they really have no justification. Unless you treat them casually, you can move into blame and recrimination.

You find happiness only within yourself. When you have found that in yourself, other people just amplify it. If you can maintain the happiness inside of you when others turn off the happiness on the outside, then you are not dependent on them for your happiness.

If you're looking for some outer form of happiness from something someone else does, what will happen to you when that other person is no longer there to do it for you? What are you going to do when you close your door at night and you are by yourself, with no one to entertain you? You can go into the depths of despair, or you can say, "It doesn't matter. I can be happy inside myself and think of beautiful things. I can redecorate my room. I'll start with the color I'd like to paint it." You start consciously directing your mind and thinking happy thoughts.

The emotions are still there, however. While you are thinking happy thoughts on one level, the emotions are sabotaging you and saying, "I've been rejected. That person doesn't love me. What if he doesn't come home? He should have been home a long time ago." You must direct your emotions, too, and this can be difficult. You have to convince yourself that the person who is out late really does love you.

You might take a flower and superstitiously pluck the petals, saying, "He loves me, he loves me not." If you end with "he loves me not," you think it's a divine omen, and you really let him have it when he comes in the door. If it ends with "he loves me," you doubt that and let him have it anyway. Sound familiar?

So many times, because of little day-to-day situations, the person you love starts becoming "the enemy." Who is really the enemy? When you do something not too intelligent and get caught, who is the enemy?

You, or the one who noticed what was going on? It's important to be honest about these things. It's also important that, after you and your loved one have told each other where to go, you remember to tell each other, "I love you." It might not be "I love you" as husband or wife, but "I love you" because of the Spirit within you, because you are an extension of God's Light, and because I can bypass the personality level that causes misunderstanding.

Levels of Loving

There are many levels of loving. One is sexual love. If two people marry based upon sexual love, the marriage will probably last six to eight weeks, until the honeymoon is over. They might get an annulment based upon incompatibility because the relationship was based only upon the man placing his body inside the woman's to see what would happen. They found out what happened, and that's all there was to it.

If the love is based upon the physical, there are more variables to consider. Let's say that you marry a person for certain physical attributes; maybe it's a 36-22-36 figure or broad shoulders and a trim waist. Those physical attributes may start to change after about a year of not chasing around, not keeping yourself trim, and watching a lot of television because, after all, you're not that interested in sex anymore. Good sex can keep you trim because the energy exchange will help balance you. If your sexual activity starts to drop off, you may move into areas that are substitutes for the sex pattern.

Two common substitutes for sex are food and alcohol; both quiet the lower self. You may sit around at night, drink two or three beers, eat some pretzels, and then go to bed. With this eating pattern, food goes to fat rapidly. If you continue this for a year, you may end up with a noticeable potbelly. Your spouse may take a look at you and think, "My God, I married you? Someone else down the street has what I'm after." Then your spouse is out traveling, going to the gym, working off the excess, getting in shape, getting sexy—for someone else. A marriage based on physical attraction can last about a year.

If the marriage is based on emotions as well as physical and sexual attraction, you will have certain feelings in common. You may both like to watch the sunset or listen to the same music. As long as the emotional quality is there, you don't need a lot of physical and sexual love. If one of you changes your attitude, however, the emotions may no longer match. She may say, "I don't care for sunsets; I'd rather watch the sunrise."

He might reply, "I don't like sunrises because I like to sleep in."

She says, "Then you sleep in with somebody else and I'll rise with someone else."

An emotional marriage can usually last about two to three years. If you can't talk to each other, however, it can become pretty dull. After three years or so of watching the sun rise and set and listening to Bach, one of you may say, "Did you like the way they played that concerto?" If the other says, "Huh?" you may start feeling mentally lonely.

That is one of the most hellish feelings, short of feeling spiritually shut off. You can go for a long time without sex, emotions, or physical bodies around you. In fact, a lot of times you want to get away from these areas. You'll go somewhere quiet to get away from people. If you can't talk to your spouse about the things you're interested in, however, it can get lonely.

Suppose one partner is studying Krishna Consciousness and the other is following Jesus. They may not be able to communicate and share mentally. When there is no mental understanding, loneliness starts coming in. This is why several churches emphasize the mind; they've had enough experience to recognize its importance.

If you can communicate mentally, the marriage can last a lifetime. As long as you can feel similar things emotionally, as long as the body is not where you're placing all your attention, and as long as you can periodically exchange sexual energy, the marriage can last a lifetime. More likely than not, it will last until the children are old enough to be on their own. Then the parents may get divorced.

The point is that the length of marriages based upon sexual, physical, emotional, or mental love is generally limited. These are all marriages of the negative realms. Marriages based on spiritual love, however, can last for eternities.

Spiritual Responsibility

It is important to maintain your identity and individuality, even when you are involved in a close personal relationship with another human being. Perhaps it is especially important then. You don't have to try to be anything you're not. You don't have to do things anyone else's way. You don't have to be like anyone else. If you realize that you can be you, then it's easy.

You may say, "Who am I?" Sometimes "I" has gotten so wrapped up with "you" that you don't know what to do. So you start cutting yourself loose. The husband may come to the wife and say, "Honey, I think you should have some outside interests and get out of the house more."

So the wife says, "Fine, I'll go to a seminar tonight."

Then he says, "No, don't go there."

She says, "Then how about the bridge club?"

He says, "Not that either. They don't do anything constructive." These are patterns of control.

As soon as you start trying to breathe other people's air for them, you'll find that you can get sick. When you are shut off from Spirit, you can become very sick physically, emotionally, and mentally. You may go to the doctor, who gives you medication to build you up so that you are physically strong enough to withstand more emotional and mental difficulties. You might be walking around in a beautiful, well-built body that is sick inside.

Then you might go to a psychologist or do some other form of therapy to work out your emotions. You come out feeling fantastic, except that your mind is still causing difficulty. It keeps going back over that same "tune," the one you dislike so much, the one you sang to that other girl or that other boy at some other time.

So, you may decide to go to a psychiatrist, who eventually gets that all straightened out for you, and you return to your loved one. Then you are content, except that there is something missing. You have fulfilled the letter of the law, but you've missed the Spirit.

Spiritual Love

You will not experience fulfillment until you can look at another person and not only say but mean, "I love you. I just love you. It doesn't matter what you do. You can't change my love. If I never see you again, I'll still love you." This is love instead of being in love.

As soon as someone says, "I'm in love with you," tell that person to back off and not come any closer, for they may want to blackmail you emotionally, mentally, and physically in order to stay in love with you. Then you'll have to do things their way. If you are just starting to stand on your own feet, it may be rough at times. You may wobble and shake a bit, but at least you're doing it on your own. If someone wants to give you a crutch to lean on, don't accept it. If you fall, you fall. You can always get back up again. If someone loves you, don't let them get in the way of your growth.

When you do something yourself, you know it's done right. If somebody else does it, that person never does it quite right. People come to me and ask me to do certain things on the physical level for them. I say, "No, you do that. I'll hold the Light and pray for you. I'll sustain you spiritually. I'll do all these things of a spiritual nature, but I will not make your decisions in this physical world. You make them."

You may worry about failing, but remember that if you fail, you get another chance. If you're afraid of failure, then do nothing. Because it's hard to do nothing, go ahead and make the best decision possible, and move forward based upon that decision.

Whatever you decide will be all right with me because I love you more than what you are deciding. If you make a decision and start moving in that direction and then think maybe you made the wrong choice, go ahead and change it. That's no problem. You can reevaluate things at any time and make new decisions based upon new information. Don't ask other people to make your decisions for you; make your own. Don't expect other people to make you happy; make your own happiness. Then you'll be shining forth the spiritual love.

Spiritual love is much like the love of parents for their baby. They may be late in leaving to visit the relatives, when the baby dirties its diaper. As parents, they have a couple of choices: either they can take the baby in its dirty diaper and misrepresent it, or they can take time and change the diaper. You know that they'll take time and change the diaper. They might not love what the baby did, but they do love that baby. That's the love I'm talking about.

Those parents might get another test if they arrive at the relatives' house and find that the baby needs its diaper changed again. One time somebody handed me a baby and said, "You won't believe this, but before we came over it was 'fix-up time,' and we get here and find out it's 'fix-up time' again."

I said, "Do you think I'm going to let a little thing like that stand between me and love? I've learned in other existences to sit on the garbage pile to eat my lunch. I can direct my mind and consciousness anywhere I wish it to be, and I wish it to be love toward this child." Loving this child was easy for me, and it was easy to take the baby, change her diaper, and clean her up. That was easy because there was love there, and nothing else could get in the way.

I've had opportunities to be in homes and watch this spiritual love manifest. The husband and wife enjoy each other sexually, they take good care of their bodies, they're moderate in their emotions, they can talk about the many things they have in common, and each one allows the other the freedom to follow his or her interests even if some don't happen to be in common.

It works like this: "If you want to go fishing today, go ahead. I'd rather sit home and read." So he goes fishing and she stays home. Later, neither one says, "You went and left me alone. You don't love me." They have a spiritual love that transcends the negative levels. In that spiritual love, they can sit together in the same room for hours, never say a word, and be totally loving.

I've watched this. I once visited some friends of mine and after dinner he began reading his sports magazine, and she started crocheting an afghan. I said, "Well, I guess I'll go home."

They said, "Wouldn't you like to spend the night?"

I said, "Doing what? I don't care to learn to crochet, and I'm not too interested in sports magazines."

They said, "Would you like to play cards or Chinese checkers? Would you like a snack?"

In other words, they were going out of their way to please me. So I said, "You're going out of your way to make me feel comfortable. I am comfortable. I just thought I'd go home, that's all. But if I can spend the night, I'd like to start spending it right now. Where am I going to be sleeping?"

They said, "We have a bed prepared in the back room for you. We just thought that since you came in from a long distance, you'd like to spend the evening with us."

I said, "That's absolutely true. I'd really love to spend the evening with you."

They said, "Okay. When you're ready to go to bed, it's just down the hall."

So while those two sat, one reading and one crocheting, I just sat there and admired them and the love that they had for each other. Their marriage was not only spiritually perfect but it was also mentally, emotionally, physically, and sexually perfect.

Some people think that sex is no longer a consideration when a person is in their sixties or seventies, but that is not so. Life doesn't necessarily begin at forty; it begins whenever you want. Age doesn't matter. People have often asked me what I think is the best age to be. My answer is always the same: "The one I am right now." That's the spiritual eternity. We all know the body will grow considerably older, but the expression of love does not have to fade with age, and the sexual expression can remain a part of that.

The important thing to understand is that when sex is expressed in love and Light, nothing else is of any consequence. If sex is expressed out of lust, you'll feel lust tomorrow. If it's expressed out of guilt, you'll feel rejected and remorseful. You may have to experience those feelings until you can clear the pattern and understand the reality of it. If you're going to have a sexual encounter, enjoy it. If you're not going to enjoy it all the way, then don't do it. It's just that simple.

Discovering Your Divinity

Sex is an experience that most everyone will be involved with one way or another. There can be favorable experiences and ones that are not so favorable. If you're smart, you'll move from those that are unfavorable to those that are uplifting, that give you fulfillment and a good feeling about yourself.

When you walk away from another person feeling as if God has blended you in an honest exchange of love, it's been a good experience. That doesn't mean that it has to be tender and gentle; it can be humorous or rough-and-tumble if that matches your disposition. It's simple: it's doing the things that work for you. Common sense is a form of spiritual awareness.

No other person and no book can tell you all you want to know about what goes on within you. There will always be questions. Sometimes, if you will be quiet long enough, you can close your eyes, drop back inside, and ask yourself, "Does this really matter in my spiritual progression and upliftment?" The question will usually disappear. It doesn't need to be answered because it isn't important. Life is very, very simple. It is to be experienced. You are to learn from your experiences and grow into greater and greater areas of awareness.

There are so many books by so many people with so many different points of view. I suppose that the books on sex would fill a library, and each one deals with the same parts of the body that we all have. It's nothing unusual; expressing sexually is natural and goes with having a physical body. There are a lot of things that go with having a physical body: getting food stuck in your teeth, catching cold, and washing the clothes. They're all part of this physical level. Are you going to attack or crucify people because of these things? Yet, if you give people a vision of their divinity, they may try to crucify you. It's happened before.

Masters have said, "You are divine; you are an extension of God." They have found that someone usually attempts to discount what they say, even though they speak the truth. Don't be foolish. Learn from the masters. Discover for yourself that you are divine. Run the assumption that there is something within you that is much more than a body.

I can prove to you that you are more than the body. Close your eyes and take a deep breath. Let it out and breathe normally. Let your body be quiet. If you have an ache, forget it for now. Let the physical pressures drop away. Now let your emotions move away from you. If you've had your feelings hurt, let that hurt go. You don't need it. Now let the mind go. Think of nothing. Let all these levels drop away. Who's doing this? When you stop moving around physically, when you drop the emotions and become calm, when you stop the mind, who is left? It's not your emotions, your mind or your body. What is left is you.

The more you come into yourself and bypass the periphery of your consciousness, the closer you will come to a place where there is a great void, a great feeling of emptiness and nothingness. You may think, "I'm getting nowhere; I'll give up." Don't do it. The Soul is protected by an etheric shield, which is the unconscious or subconscious area of your consciousness; it can be dark and void. When you endure past that, you break into the awareness of God. Then, while you reside within the physical, emotional, mental, and unconscious bodies, your consciousness resides in paradise, or heaven. At this point, you will know that you are divine and that you are the Beloved. You'll know that Alpha and Omega are names that also apply to you—not to you as your physical body, but to you as your Soul.

The spiritual path is easy; it is the only path there is. It's difficult when you attempt to separate yourself from the spiritual. Then you experience confusion, upset, and turmoil. When you experience these difficulties, it is God indicating through Spirit that you have stepped from the reality of your true self. When you come back into the oneness of Spirit, you find out that the blessings already are. All that you want to be, you already are. All you have to do is move your awareness there and recognize the reality of your own Soul.

Bibliography of Books & Tapes by John-Roger

Items are audio tapes unless otherwise noted. V preceding a number denotes the tape is also available in video format. SAT stands for Soul Awareness Tapes, which are audio tapes of John-Roger's seminars, meditations, and sharings that are sent each month only to SAT subscribers. Once you subscribe, you can obtain previously issued tapes. Please note that some of the tapes in this Bibliography are SAT tapes, and you would need to subscribe to the series to order them.

The Age of Getting (#1127)
Can a Marriage Be Threatened? (#2626)
How Do You Overcome Violence? (#7503, #V-7503)
How Guilt is Built and its Effects (#1704)

Keeping Relationships Wholly/Holy (#4011)

Live the Principles of Your Experiences (#7405, #V-7405)

Psychic Violence (#7308, #V-7308)

Psychic-Sexual Energies (#3208)

The Power Struggle Game (#2141)

Relationships, Initiation, Restoration and Consequences (#7656, #V-7656)

Relationships: Love, Marriage and Spirit (Book, available in bookstores everywhere, ISBN #0-893020-05-3)

Sexual-Spiritual Responsibilities & Hoo Chant (#2055)

Shame: Does God See Us? (#7497, #V-7497)

Spiritual Warrior, The Art of Spiritual Success (Book, available in bookstores everywhere, ISBN 0-914829-36-X)

Spiritual Warrior/El Guerrero Espiritual (#7333, #V-7333)

Social - Sexual Behavior (#7186, SAT Tape)

The Spiritual Marriage (#2105)

The Spiritual Family (Book, available in bookstores everywhere, ISBN #0-914829-21-1)

Submission, Sex, and Soul Awareness (#2139)

The Traveler and Balancing Left and Right-Sided Energies (#7432, SAT Tape)

Thoughts, Consciousness, and Manifestation (#7072)

Upgrade Your Addictions to God (#7487, SAT Tape)

Other - Ongoing Spiritual Study

MSIA on the Internet at http://www.msia.org

The web site offers a free subscription to MSIA's daily inspirational e-mail, Loving Each Day; the *New Day Herald* on-line; the opportunity to request that names be placed on the prayer list; MSIA's catalog, and much more.

Soul Awareness Discourses
If you like this book, Discourses are a gold mine of further information, as well as a resource for a deeper connection with Spirit. Here is a sample of the contents: highest good in Discourses 2 and 109; communication in Discourse 99; discipline in Discourses 44 and 77; speaking kind words in Discourse 50; three selves in Discourse 17; and much more. (Twelve books per year, one for each month, English, Spanish, or French, #5000).

Soul Awareness Tape (SAT) Series
A new JohnRoger seminar every month, plus access to the entire SAT library of hundreds of meditations & seminars. (Twelve tapes per year, one per month, #5400)

Soul Journey through Spiritual Exercises
    (Three tape album with booklet; #3718)
Spiritual Exercises: Walking with the Lord
    (Four tape album, #3907)

Books by John-Roger
Available through bookstores everywhere

Divine Essence ISBN 1-893020-04-5
Forgiveness, The Key to the Kingdom ISBN 0-914829-62-9
Inner Worlds of Meditation ISBN 0-914829-45-9
Loving Each Day ISBN 0-914829-26-2
Manual on Using the Light ISBN 0-914829-13-0
The Path to Mastership ISBN 0-914829-16-5
The Power Within You ISBN 0-914829-24-6
The Tao of Spirit ISBN 0-914829-33-5

Tapes and books are available from:
MSIA®
P.O. Box 513935
Los Angeles, CA 90051
323-737-4055 FAX 323-737-5680
jrbooks@msia.org
http://www.mandevillepress.org

Books are available at Borders, Barnes & Noble, many
independent bookstores, and amazon.com.

About John-Roger

A teacher and lecturer of international stature, with millions of books in print, John-Roger has helped people to discover the Spirit within themselves and find health, peace, and prosperity for over three decades.

With two co-authored books on the *New York Times* Best-Seller List, and more than three dozen books and audio albums, John-Roger is an extraordinary resource on many subjects. He is the founder of the nondenominational Church of the Movement of Spiritual Inner Awareness (MSIA) which focuses on Soul Transcendence; President of the Institute for Individual and World Peace; Chancellor of the University of Santa Monica; and President of Peace Theological Seminary & College of Philosophy.

John-Roger has given over 5,000 seminars world-
wide, many of which are televised nationally on his
cable program, "That Which Is." He has been a fea-
tured guest on the "Roseane Show," "Politically
Incorrect," and CNN's "Larry King Live," and
appears regularly on radio and television.

An educator and minister by profession, John-Roger
continues to work from his hometown of Los Angeles,
California to transform the lives of many by educating
them in the wisdom of the spiritual heart.